Reversing Rabies Virus: Deficiencies

The Raw Vegan Plant-Based Detoxification & Regeneration Workbook for Healing Patients.

Volume 4

I0090496

Health Central

Copyright © 2023

Topics Discussed & Journal Structure

Points Discussed in Volume 3

1 – Why do we experience cravings and how to manage them (and which herbs to use)?

2 – Understanding the biology of the gut.

3 – The cleansing nature of fruit sugar (Fructose).

4 – Satisfying raw vegan foods proven to curb that cravings urge if and when it comes.

5 – Forming new habits through a dietary transition phase.

6 – Supporting emotional imbalances and habitual/comfort eating.

7 – The best gift you could give to yourself and your health.

Deficiencies & Absorption

"DEFICIENCIES are to blame…" says Mr Porter (Dietician) to his patient, Albert.

For argument's sake let's assume that the dietician is correct, and that deficiencies are to blame for Albert's sickness. Could it then be due to Albert's food being deficient in nutrition? He eats a variety of foods daily, including fresh fruits and vegetables, but yet he is still "deficient" in all the main vitamins and minerals. How could this be?

Many professionals from within the health sector offer questionable dietary advice to patients ("eat more meat for protein" or "take Chromium for your Pancreas"). Sadly this advice is based on a misguided premise – with treatment and symptom management (and not the cure) being the goal.

If you are advised that your conditions are due solely to deficiencies then you are not being presented with the complete picture - because if indeed you are deficient, there is a deeper issue at play. If you are eating foods that are loaded with vitamins and minerals but yet you are still low on them – it is easy to be misled into thinking that your diet is unhealthy.

However we should first look at the root causes and their related factors. The foundation stone of your body is its terrain. So for

example if the processes of digestion, absorption, utilisation, and healthy elimination of your waste are hindered, this will eventually create problems for you. In order to correct absorption issues, we must first understand how the lymphatic system works. Additionally, an understanding of utilisation is necessary. Without these tools, you will risk remaining constipated (both mentally and physically) whilst ignoring the causative factors of your health challenges.

Now that we understand that everything stems from the terrain of your body, our focus is turned towards removing the congested sewage that blocks the flow of energy in relation to eliminating effectively. The removal of damaging acid from the body is vital for your key organs and glands to recover and resume utilisation of the consumed nutrition, vitamins and minerals.

All too often we find the small intestines of our patients to be interstitially (deep within cells and tissues) damaged with acids, and their large intestines (and colon) are plastered with mucoid plaque. This is the root cause of poor absorption of nutrition and this means that you will not receive the full benefits from your consumed foods. This also means that taking supplements will not necessarily yield the results that you desire. Instead, they could potentially worsen the issue and over-stimulate and acidify your body.

Cleanse Your Lymphatic System: Your lymphatic system needs to be flushed out in order for your absorption and utilisation to start working for you again. This sewage system is your body's main elimination backbone, and is responsible for cleansing your blood and organs of accumulated acids and waste.

Acids damage the soft tissue infrastructure within your body. If the foods that you consume are acidic, regardless of them being full of "nutrition", you will continue to suffer from cell damage and a breakdown of your eliminative organs (kidneys, bowels, skin, lungs). This will lead to waste backing up within your different systems, which will cause damage to organs such as the adrenal glands which are responsible for mineral utilisation.

Your adrenal glands also work hand-in-hand with the kidneys, and with the adrenal glands struggling, your kidneys also risk losing their ability to effectively filter and remove the acids out of your lymphatic system.

As you can see, your body is built up of an interconnected system which needs to be corrected systemically. We want to target the root causes by cleansing the body's sewage clearing system, correct digestion, absorption, utilization and eliminate accumulated metabolic waste, along with any hidden old faecal matter waste from previous poor dietary habits. We also need to remove mucus through our eliminative organs whilst also removing the destructive acids that are responsible for breaking down tissues, which effectively leads to internal dysfunction, imbalance and eventual dis-ease within the body.

How? We must start by becoming conscious and aware of the destructive foods that we are actively eating on a daily basis. All cooked foods with their energy sapping nature, along with the added chemicals which cause damage to your organs, and central and autonomic nervous systems - must be removed from your routine.

You will also need to remove the following from your day-to-day lifestyle in order to make positive healing gains:

a) Genetically Modified Organisms (GMOs) – e.g. corn, soy.

b) All neurotoxic pesticide-immersed foods – but in the case of fruits typically high in pesticides (strawberries, nectarines, apples, grapes, peaches, cherries, etc) – we leave them soaking in baking soda and warm water for 15 minutes before washing off.

c) All chemical-based skin products - and breathable toxic chemicals (e.g. hair sprays, deodorant).

d) Fluoride water used for drinking and bathing in (use a filter instead).

e) Eliminate the combined consumption of wheat and animal products - it is these that contribute mostly towards disturbing your absorption and utilisation.

A variety of acidic and sub-acidic fruits, including berries, melons, citrus, will all promote the cleansing of your lymphatic system, and support you in opening up your eliminative organs and related endocrine glands. We MUST make a gradual transition from your current diet (by eliminating the dehydrating foods) and start introducing a raw fruit-based diet which is hydrating, cleansing and full of biologically available nutrition for your cells. With any transition, the secret is to support your adrenal glands, kidneys, and digestive organs.

When you finally start absorbing effectively, you will find that you actually do not require large portions in order to feel strong and full of energy.

If at the extreme end of sickness - we have recommended moving into a full slow-juiced fruit regimen, incorporating herbal and glandular formulas. Herbs and glandular formulas will support you in transitioning over from a previous diet as it can be quite a shock and stressful for the body when moving over to a fully raw diet. Vegetable juices (e.g. juiced carrots, celery, beetroots) will also support you through this phase.

Helpful Notes: The subject of transitioning over from a standard diet to a raw fruit and vegetable diet is a delicate one and if not done correctly, you will experience some challenges. However, this is normal because considering that your body is congested from your regular dietary routine – to now having a detoxifying diet will mean that your body will send out a variety of signals due to it no longer being fed what it had become accustomed to.

During this phase of transition, based on experience with our patients, we recommend that you support the following organs:

1. The Pituitary Gland (PG) stimulates its fellow endocrine glands (Thyroid, Parathyroid, Adrenal, Pancreas, Gonads, Pineal). So if the PG is down – the other related glands will also likely be suffering. In order to support the PG, we typically use small amounts of pituitary glandular formula concentrations for chronic patients, and herbs (tincture form being preferred initially) that promote healthy brain and nerve blood circulation (e.g. Gingko, Hawthorn Berry). For dosage information, you must start off small and work up to what feels comfortable for you.

2. The Parathyroid Gland regulates calcium utilization. For effective calcium uptake into the body, and strong bones, we need to

ensure that the calcium that we are consuming from food is being put to work otherwise there will be an imbalance and the stagnant acids in your lymphatic system will pinch the calcium from your bones, resulting in weaker bones (and varicose veins, brain herniation, anxiety, depression, spider veins, brittle fingernails, low calcium levels, bone spurs, fibroids, hemorrhoids, osteoporosis, scoliosis, arthritis, prolapsing of organs).

For optimal parathyroid function, we must ensure that the lymphatic system is being flushed out of acids through a high fruit regimen, whilst maintaining a decent level of calcium through the diet. The herbs Horsetail and Alfalfa are rich in calcium. We have found sea moss to also be effective for overall bone health.

3. The Adrenal Glands (sat right on top of your kidneys) are responsible for sugar metabolisation and mineral utilisation. These glands are yet another set of organs that we find patients

to be struggling with. When moving over to a high fruit diet, the adrenal glands can struggle to cope with the high levels of sugar. This can result in weight gain, specifically around the girth and waist area due to the body's desire to protect its vital organs and glands. You will also find that the change in diet will cause a slight stress response from your adrenal glands, which can then lead to many additional symptoms – a common one being an increased salt craving. However, you must continue to push forward as this will be short-lived because a high fruit diet will flush out your whole urinary tract, including your adrenal glands and kidneys. To address salt cravings, we have previously found coconut water and juiced celery to help.

Some of the herbs that we found to be useful in supporting the adrenal glands include Parsley, Kelp, Licorice Root, Cleavers, Saw Palmetto, Dandelion Root.

4. Your Kidneys (including your skin – the 3rd kidney) are the most important eliminative organs within your lymphatic system. The acidic lymph waste will leave your body through these avenues, so it is crucial that we are taking care of them. Again, a hydrating and cleansing high fruit diet will help to wash out your kidneys, and the addition of herbs will support your progress. Some of the herbs that we use for improving kidney health include: Uva Ursi, Parsley, and Stinging Nettle Leaf. Remember to also keep up water intake with Spring Water being the preferred type.

5. Intestines/Colon – many recommend enemas and colonics and although we are not opposed to these practices every so often, we prefer to focus on our methodology of improving health from within (the cellular level). Besides fruits such as grapes, mangos, prunes, figs – the herbs that we use to support a deep gut cleanse include Cascara Sagrada (gentle laxative) and Slippery Elm Bark (for lubrication of the gut).

6. Physical activities to perform that we have found to aide lymphatic cleansing include:

a) Sweating with a sauna or in a hot climate helps with the elimination of acids.

b) Raising vitamin D levels naturally through exposure to sunlight also contributes towards healing.

c) Deep breathing exercises by the sea (or any other "off-grid" fresh environment) are vital for the acceleration of your healing. Oxygen has a huge part to play in good health and the deterrence of dis-ease. We learnt many invaluable breathing techniques and practices off Wim Hof. You are welcome to research his work and apply it to yourself.

d) If you are able to do so, jumping on the rebounder/trampoline has been found to help mobilize a stagnant lymphatic fluid whilst offering great cardiovascular benefits. Start off slow - jumping for as long as is comfortable and work up to 15 to 20 minutes per day. As you progress and grow in confidence, you can try out different jumping techniques.

If these activities listed in point 6 are not possible due to your circumstances – we would recommend staying active on a daily basis at the very least – and sweat where possible.

Finally... Our goal is to remove acids from your body whilst hydrating and alkalizing it. A fruit diet, with some vegetables from time to time, combined with intermittent dry fasting is the way to achieve this. Let's tackle the root causes and empower our health to a frequency of high vibration and electricity so our bodies normalise and become dis-ease free.

Good luck – stay focused – remain persistent – visualize your successes – you WILL achieve your desired goals. Wishing you the best of health. Good luck with your healing journey.

Our Story

It was a Sunday night, over 7 years ago – I was in bed – tossing and turning – unable to sleep. I watched the time pass, from 11pm, to 12am… to 1:30am. I just couldn't sleep. I could feel an immense pressure in my chest cavity and all across my diaphragm area. I couldn't understand where this was coming from. I got up and had some water, I then tried to use the bathroom – the discomfort was still there. Nothing seemed to work – I felt like I was being suffocated each time I would lie down. In the end, I fell asleep out of sheer fatigue.

At the time, I was a sufferer of asthma, eczema, anxiety attacks, and a damaged/leaky gut. These conditions had lead to many symptoms that doctors could not offer me any answers for. I had many tests done but nothing could tell me what the root causes of my problems were.

I started researching about my symptoms, and as I did this, I found myself expanding into the area of medical history. As my research continued, I came to understand that our ancestors lived healthy and long lives, without the health challenges of today.

Eventually, I stumbled upon a few health forums which I joined. Through these, I met a series of individuals that were battling a variety of conditions themselves (a rare genetic disorder, Crohn's disease, multiple sclerosis, muscular dystrophy (MD), diabetes, cushing's disease, a series of 'incurable' autoimmune diseases, and cancer).

We all came together and as we started to grow as a group, we made a significant discovery - that actually the cure to all diseases was discovered back in the 1920s by a Dr Arnold Ehret.

As we studied his material, we started applying his information and protocols on ourselves. This seemed like one experiment worth trying, and within 2 weeks, regardless of our individual conditions, we all started to notice a difference in our improved digestion, higher energy levels, increased mental clarity and improved physical ability. A major change was taking place – our health was improving, as our conditions were decreasing.

We continued to expand our knowledge and we started to encounter even more communities and learnt that there were more magnificent and very gifted healers out there. We came across the works and achievements of Dr Sebi, and completed an insightful and very informative course by Dr Robert Morse.

The essential message of these great healers was very similar to that of Dr Arnold Ehret. Now we had even further confirmation that the information we had been following thus far was in fact THE path to health success. With our progress so far, we could sense victory.

Within 3 months, 30 to 40 percent of our symptoms had disappeared and our health was becoming stronger. Some of us started to take specific herbs in order to enhance the detoxification.

Another 3 months on and the majority of us no longer experienced any more symptoms. Our blood work had also improved significantly, but we still had work to do in order to completely heal.

Now that we had made significant progress in reversing our conditions through self-experimentation, we started to offer basic healthy eating advice to the sick within our local communities.

Eventually, we started working with local patients on a voluntary basis. It was heartbreaking to witness lives being cut short or chronic sickness being accepted as a way of life – all whilst the lifelong eating habits of these individuals remained. The most common diseases that we were coming across included: cancers, heart disease, chronic kidney disease, high blood pressure, varying infections, and diabetes.

By helping our communities with changing their daily eating habits, we started seeing results, and although the transitional phase of moving from the foods that they were so used to eating, to moving over to a raw plant-based routine was a challenge, in the end, it was worth the shift. Note: there were many that ignored our advice and sadly they continued to remain in their state.

We did have resistance initially from family members and friends of the sick but after some time as they started seeing health improvements, more started joining us, and they also started experiencing what we had when we first set out on our journey of natural self-healing.

Nevertheless, challenges still remained – the main ones being the undoing of society's programming that cooked food is an essential part of life (including animal and wheat based products) and raw food alone surely cannot be good for you. It doesn't take long to explain how to remove imbalances and dis-ease from within the human body but the more extensive task is to actually have the protocol information applied and adhered to completely.

This is where the idea for this series of journal & progress tracker stemmed from. We felt compelled to spread this information in a more digestible and applicable form, over a series of volumes, in which we would start by offering some key informative points, followed by a journal which would allow for you to actually apply the information, record your progress, daily feelings and stay accountable to yourself. We also found that journaling and writing to oneself really helps to self-motivate and enhances a self consciousness that is needed when following a protocol like this.

Each journal volume within this series will be designed to help you record your journey for a 30 day period. At the start of each journal we will continue to offer insightful information about our experiences, whilst expanding on and re-iterating specific parts of this protocol.

The fact that you are reading this foreword is an indication that you are already on your way to self-healing. Regardless of your condition, we invite you to seek more knowledge and set your health free.

May you always remain blessed and guided.

Much Love From The Health Central Team

Important Notes for Overcoming Your Rabies Virus

1. It should be noted that based on our experiences and understanding, whether your condition is Rabies Virus, or any other, we recommend the same raw vegan healing protocol across all spectrums. With some conditions, you may need to perform a deeper detoxification (using herbs - or organ/glandular meat/capsules for more chronic situations) before achieving significant results, but in general, we have found this protocol to work in most cases. In our experience, the goal is not to cure, but instead to raise health levels first, through healthy food choices, as intended for our species – before the eradication and prevention of these modern-day "disease" conditions can take place.

2. With all conditions, we have found that the lymphatic system has become congested and overwhelmed due to the kidneys not efficiently filtering out the accumulated cell waste – as a result of years of dehydrating cooked/wheat/dairy foods. The adrenal glands work closely with the kidneys, and so adrenal/kidney herbs and glandular formulas played a major role in opening up these channels. We also found that opening up the bowels and loosening the gut was hugely important too.

3. The healing protocol that we used on ourselves is discussed and expanded upon throughout the various volumes in this series. Our goal is to share information that we have gathered from our journeys, and let you decide if it is something that you feel could also work for you in your

journey for health and vitality. You are not obliged to use this information, and you may proceed as you see fit.

Through our study, research and application, we have found this system to correct any internal imbalances and remove dis-ease that has occurred within the human body, due to the continued consumption of acid-forming foods.

4. Always take progression ultra slow and go at your own pace. Listen to your body at every stage. We cannot re-iterate this point enough. Pay attention to how you feel and continue to consult your doctor and monitor your blood work.

5. A special emphasis needs to be given to the transition phase when moving from your regular, standard diet, to a raw vegan diet that is high in fruit. You must take your time and slowly remove foods from your current routine, and replace them with either fasting or a small amount of fruit in the initial stages. Work with small amounts – please do not make any drastic changes. If you do not feel comfortable or have any concerns at any stage, please immediately stop.

Note: with any dietary change, this can be a stressful event for the body and so it is important that you support your kidneys and adrenal glands using the appropriate herbs and glandular formulas previously mentioned.

6. Before partaking in any new dietary routine, please always consult your Doctor first and ensure that they are aware of your health related goals. This approach is beneficial because (a) you can monitor your blood work with your doctor as you progress with this new protocol, and (b) if you are on any medication, as your health improves, you

can review its need and/or discuss having dosage amounts reduced (if necessary).

7. Please note that we are sharing information from our collective experiences of how we healed ourselves from a variety of diseases and conditions. These are solely our own opinions. Having reversed a range of conditions using essentially the same protocol, our understanding and conclusion, based on our experience alone, is that regardless of the disease, illness or condition name – removing it from the human body stems from correcting your diet and transitioning over to a more raw vegan lifestyle.

8. Proceed with care, and again, do not make any sudden changes – always take your time in slowly removing foods that are not serving you, and replacing them with high energy sweet tree-ripened juicy fruit. If at any point you feel that you are moving too quickly, please adjust your transition accordingly. Results may vary between individuals.

9. We recommended that you constantly expand your knowledge and familiarise yourself with the works of Dr Arnold Ehret, Dr Robert Morse and John Rose. When you feel confident with your understanding, start taking gradual steps towards reaching your goals. Make the most of this journal and use it to serve you as a companion on your journey.

The Power of Journaling

a) Journaling your inner self talk is a truly effective way of increasing self awareness and consciousness. To be able to transfer your thoughts and feelings onto a piece of paper is a truly effective method of self reflection and improvement. This is much needed when you are switching to a high fruit dietary routine.

b) Be sure to always add the date of journaling at the top of each page used. This is invaluable for when you wish to go back and review/track progress and your feelings/thoughts on previous dates.

c) Keep a comprehensive record of activities, thoughts, and really log everything you ate/are eating. You can even make miscellaneous notes if you feel that they will help you.

d) We have added tips and questions to offer you guidance, reminders, inspiration and areas to journal about.

e) We like to use journals to have a conversation with ourselves. Inner talk can really help you overcome any challenges that you are experiencing. Express yourself and any concerns that you may have.

f) Try to advise yourself as though you are your best friend – similarly to how you would advise a close friend or family member. You will be surprised at the results that you will achieve from using this technique.

g) Add notes to this journal and work your way through the 30 days. Once completed, move onto the next journal volume in this series, which will also be structured in a similar, supportive and educational fashion. We have produced a series of these journals in order to cater for your ongoing journey and goals.

h) For those of you who would like to track your progress with a more basic notebook-style journal, we have produced a separate series in which each notebook interior differs. This is to cater for your complete health journaling needs.

We have laid out the following examples to serve as potential frameworks for one way of how a journal could be filled in on a daily basis. These are just basic examples, but you can complete your daily journals in any other way that you feel is most comfortable and effective for you.

[EXAMPLE 1]

Today's Date: 2nd Jan 2020

Morning

I just ate 3 mangoes - very sweet and tasty. I felt a heavy feeling under my chest area so I stopped eating. Unsure what that was - maybe digestive or the transverse colon?

Afternoon

I was feeling hungry so I am eating some dried figs, pineapple and apricots with around 750ml of spring water.

Evening

Sipping on a green tea (herbal). Feeling pretty strong and alert at the moment.

Night

Enjoying a bowl of red seeded grapes. Currently I feel satisfied.

Today's Notes (Highlights, Thoughts, Feelings):

Unlike yesterday, today was a good day. I am noticing an increase in regular bowel movements which makes me feel cleansed and light afterwards. I feel as though my kidneys are also starting to filter better (white sediment visible in morning wee).

It definitely helps to document my thoughts in this workbook. A great way to reflect, improve and stay on track.

Feeling very good - vibrant and strong - I have noticed a major improvement in my physical fitness and performance. Mentally I feel healthier and happier.

[EXAMPLE 2]
Today's Date: 3rd Jan 2020

Morning

Dry fasting (water and food free since 8pm last night) - will go up until 12:30pm today, and start with 500ml of spring water before eating half a watermelon.

Afternoon

Kept busy and was in and out quite a bit - so nothing consumed.

Evening

At around 5pm, I had a peppermint tea with a selection of mixed dried fruit (small bowl of apricot, dates, mango, pineapple, and prunes).

Night

Sipped on spring water through the evening as required.
Finished off the other half of the watermelon from the morning.

Today's Notes (Highlights, Thoughts, Feelings):

As with most days, today started well with me dry fasting (continuing my fast from my sleep/skipping breakfast) up until around 12:30pm and then eating half a watermelon. The laxative effect of the watermelon helped me poop and release any loosened toxins from the fasting period.
I tend to struggle on some days from 3pm onwards. Up until that point I am okay but if the cravings strike then it can be challenging. I remind myself that those burgers and chips do not have any live healing energy.
I feel good in general. I feel fantastic doing a fruit/juice fast but slightly empty by the end of the day.
Cooked food makes me feel severe fatigue and mental fog.
Will continue with my fruit fasting and start to introduce fruit juices due to their deeper detox benefits. I would love to be on juices only as I have seen others within the community achieve amazing results.

[EXAMPLE 3]
Today's Date: 4th Jan 2020

Morning
Today I woke and my children were enjoying some watermelon for breakfast - and the smell was luring so I joined them. Large bowl of watermelon eaten at around 8am. Started with a glass of water.

Afternoon
Snacked on left over watermelon throughout the morning and afternoon. Had 5 dates an hour or so after.

Evening
Had around 3 mangoes at around 6pm. Felt content - but then I was invited round to a family gathering where a selection of pizzas, burgers and chips were being served. I gave into the peer pressure and felt like I let myself down!

Night
Having over-eaten earlier on in the evening, I was still feeling bloated with a headache (possibly digestion related) and I also felt quite mucus filled (wheez in chest and coughing up phlegm). Very sleepy and low energy. The perils of cooked foods!!

Today's Notes (Highlights, Thoughts, Feelings):

I let myself down today. It all started well until I ate a fully blown meal (and over-ate). I didn't remain focussed and I spun off track. As a result my energy levels were much lower and I felt a bout of extreme fatigue 30 minutes after the meal (most likely the body struggling to with digesting all that cooked food).
I need to stick to the plan because the difference between fruit fasting, and eating cooked foods is huge - 1 makes you feel empowered whilst the other makes you feel drained. I also felt the mucus overload after the meal - it kicked in pretty quickly.
Today I felt disappointed after giving in to the meal but tomorrow is a new day and I will keep on going! It is important to remind myself that I won't get better if I cannot stick to the routine.

Frequently Asked Questions (Vol. 4)

1. Does dry fasting involve not showering or brushing my teeth?

Not entirely but some do take it to this level. We simply recommend that you work up towards not eating or drinking for prolonged periods (18+ hours) - ideally from the previous night until the evening before breaking your fast with dates, prune juice, grapes, oranges - or any other laxative based fruit that you enjoy. Also stay hydrated with water. We dry fast every Monday and Thursday (until dinner time). You can do what feels easiest for you.

2. What if my sodium and potassium levels drop down on a fruit diet?

Initially, going from a standard diet, your organs will not be completely prepared to respond to the full force of fruits. This is where you will need to strengthen any weak organs such as the adrenal glands, kidneys, and various digestive organs - so that absorption and utilisation can take place efficiently and your body is supported through this dietary transition. An Iris Diagnosis can also highlight your main weaknesses. We have found juiced celery and coconut water to be very supportive for sodium and potassium. You can also add in some leafy greens to your juices. Pink salt sprinkled lightly on salads helped us in the past but we prefer the more plant-based sources.

3. My friend recommended that I take part in Ramadan and fast for a whole month with her. She said I will feel more present-minded and I will have a feeling of

accountability. Is this a good idea?

Yes. Any type of prolonged dry fasting will yield beneficial results however do note that after fasting you must open with a laxative based fruit (dates, prunes, figs), followed by fruits that are kind to your kidneys (oranges, grapes, melons) and will support them through filtration. Water is also very important. With fasting, we must focus on the elimination organs (kidneys, skin, gut) because fasting itself starves off weak/damaged cells and accumulates toxins, ready for disposal. These need to be disposed of gently during the fast opening period. Additionally, any type of accountability is a good idea because it will keep you on track to reach your goals. Note: if you are fasting for the first time, ensure you are supporting your kidneys with herbs and/or glandulars. Water and hydration is another major key when it comes to dry fasting.

4. Is it true that disease starts at the colon?

I would say that to reverse a chronic condition, you must start by cleansing your lower digestive system which includes the intestines and colon. The kidneys also play a vital role in this process. We have found that the most chronic patients have one thing in common – they all have a deeply congested colon. Practicing enema cleanses every so often, drinking the cold-pressed juice of plums (or dates, grapes, prunes, oranges, figs) and taking herbs such as Cascara Sagrada, and Slippery Elm Bark have all served us well.

1. Today's Date:

Morning

(work towards continuing your night time dry fast up until at least 12pm)

Afternoon

(get hydrating with fresh fruit or even better slow juiced fruits/berries/melons)

Evening

(aim to wind down to a dry fast by around 6pm to 7pm)

Night

(work your way up to dry fasting from the evening until 12pm the following day)

Today's Notes (Highlights, Thoughts, Feelings, What Could You Improve On?)

"Get yourself an accountability partner to complete a 30 day detox with. Start with 7 days and work your way up. It will be fun and motivating completing it with somebody (or a group) ...or of course you can go it alone."

---

2. Today's Date:

Morning

(work towards continuing your night time dry fast up until at least 12pm)

Afternoon

(get hydrating with fresh fruit or even better slow juiced fruits/berries/melons)

Evening

(aim to wind down to a dry fast by around 6pm to 7pm)

Night

(work your way up to dry fasting from the evening until 12pm the following day)

Today's Notes (Highlights, Thoughts, Feelings, What Could You Improve On?)

"Remember when starting out, it is important to keep yourself hydrated throughout the day. Spring Water is a good start - and slow/cold pressed juice is also very powerful."

3. Today's Date:

Morning

(work towards continuing your night time dry fast up until at least 12pm)

Afternoon

(get hydrating with fresh fruit or even better slow juiced fruits/berries/melons)

Evening

(aim to wind down to a dry fast by around 6pm to 7pm)

Night

(work your way up to dry fasting from the evening until 12pm the following day)

Today's Notes (Highlights, Thoughts, Feelings, What Could You Improve On?)

"Eat melons/watermelons separately, and before any other fruit as it digests faster and we want to limit fermentation (acidity) which can occur if other fruits are mixed in."

4. Today's Date:

Morning
(work towards continuing your night time dry fast up until at least 12pm)

Afternoon
(get hydrating with fresh fruit or even better slow juiced fruits/berries/melons)

Evening
(aim to wind down to a dry fast by around 6pm to 7pm)

Night
(work your way up to dry fasting from the evening until 12pm the following day)

Today's Notes (Highlights, Thoughts, Feelings, What Could You Improve On?)

"Stay focussed on the end goal of removing mucus & toxins from your body and feeling wonderful! Look forward to being full of vitality and disease free once again"

5. Today's Date:

Morning

(work towards continuing your night time dry fast up until at least 12pm)

Afternoon

(get hydrating with fresh fruit or even better slow juiced fruits/berries/melons)

Evening

(aim to wind down to a dry fast by around 6pm to 7pm)

Night

(work your way up to dry fasting from the evening until 12pm the following day)

Today's Notes (Highlights, Thoughts, Feelings, What Could You Improve On?)

"Meditate and perform deep breathing exercises in order to help yourself remain present minded and on track. Perform these techniques throughout the day but also during any challenging times that you may come to face."

6. Today's Date:

Morning

(work towards continuing your night time dry fast up until at least 12pm)

Afternoon

(get hydrating with fresh fruit or even better slow juiced fruits/berries/melons)

Evening

(aim to wind down to a dry fast by around 6pm to 7pm)

Night

(work your way up to dry fasting from the evening until 12pm the following day)

Today's Notes (Highlights, Thoughts, Feelings, What Could You Improve On?)

"Join a few like-minded communities – there are many juicing and raw vegan based groups, both online and offline. Being part of a community can help motivate you to reach your goals. You will also learn a great amount from others. Seeing others succeed is empowering."

---

7. Today's Date:

Morning
(work towards continuing your night time dry fast up until at least 12pm)

Afternoon
(get hydrating with fresh fruit or even better slow juiced fruits/berries/melons)

Evening
(aim to wind down to a dry fast by around 6pm to 7pm)

Night
(work your way up to dry fasting from the evening until 12pm the following day)

Today's Notes (Highlights, Thoughts, Feelings, What Could You Improve On?)

"If you are struggling to cope with hunger
pangs in the early stages, try some dates
or dried apricots, prunes, or raisins, with
a cup of herbal tea. However, these pangs will disappear
once your body adjusts to your new routine."

8. Today's Date:

Morning
(work towards continuing your night time dry fast up until at least 12pm)

Afternoon
(get hydrating with fresh fruit or even better slow juiced fruits/berries/melons)

Evening
(aim to wind down to a dry fast by around 6pm to 7pm)

Night
(work your way up to dry fasting from the evening until 12pm the following day)

Today's Notes (Highlights, Thoughts, Feelings, What Could You Improve On?)

"Get into a routine of regularly buying fresh fruit (or grow your own if weather permits) to keep your supplies up. Local wholesale markets do also clear fruit on Fridays (if they are closed for the weekend) at a lower price, so they are worth a visit."

9. Today's Date:

Morning

(work towards continuing your night time dry fast up until at least 12pm)

Afternoon

(get hydrating with fresh fruit or even better slow juiced fruits/berries/melons)

Evening

(aim to wind down to a dry fast by around 6pm to 7pm)

Night

(work your way up to dry fasting from the evening until 12pm the following day)

Today's Notes (Highlights, Thoughts, Feelings, What Could You Improve On?)

"Regularly remind yourself about the great rewards and benefits that you will experience by keeping up this detoxification process. Imagine the lives you could save as a result of healing yourself."

10. Today's Date:

Morning

(work towards continuing your night time dry fast up until at least 12pm)

Afternoon

(get hydrating with fresh fruit or even better slow juiced fruits/berries/melons)

Evening

(aim to wind down to a dry fast by around 6pm to 7pm)

Night

(work your way up to dry fasting from the evening until 12pm the following day)

Today's Notes (Highlights, Thoughts, Feelings, What Could You Improve On?)

"Keep your teeth brushed and flossed regularly – at least twice a day (morning & night) to keep them healthy for your fruit sessions. You will notice an improvement in your dental health with this raw/fruit diet."

11. Today's Date:

Morning

(work towards continuing your night time dry fast up until at least 12pm)

Afternoon

(get hydrating with fresh fruit or even better slow juiced fruits/berries/melons)

Evening

(aim to wind down to a dry fast by around 6pm to 7pm)

Night

(work your way up to dry fasting from the evening until 12pm the following day)

Today's Notes (Highlights, Thoughts, Feelings, What Could You Improve On?)

"Be motivated by the vision of becoming an example for others to learn from and follow. You could change the lives of family and friends by showing them your own improvements."

12. Today's Date:

Morning

(work towards continuing your night time dry fast up until at least 12pm)

Afternoon

(get hydrating with fresh fruit or even better slow juiced fruits/berries/melons)

Evening

(aim to wind down to a dry fast by around 6pm to 7pm)

Night

(work your way up to dry fasting from the evening until 12pm the following day)

Today's Notes (Highlights, Thoughts, Feelings, What Could You Improve On?)

"Embrace your achievements and wonderful results – feel and appreciate the difference within you as a result of this new routine. Notice how your personal agility and fitness has improved. Feel the improved energy levels."

13. Today's Date:

Morning
(work towards continuing your night time dry fast up until at least 12pm)

Afternoon
(get hydrating with fresh fruit or even better slow juiced fruits/berries/melons)

Evening
(aim to wind down to a dry fast by around 6pm to 7pm)

Night
(work your way up to dry fasting from the evening until 12pm the following day)

Today's Notes (Highlights, Thoughts, Feelings, What Could You Improve On?)

"Buy fruit in bulk where possible so you have ample supplies for a week or two in advance. If in a hot climate, you could even freeze your fruit or make ice lollies out of it (crush & freeze). Immerse yourself in fruit so it becomes your only option."

14. Today's Date:

Morning

(work towards continuing your night time dry fast up until at least 12pm)

Afternoon

(get hydrating with fresh fruit or even better slow juiced fruits/berries/melons)

Evening

(aim to wind down to a dry fast by around 6pm to 7pm)

Night

(work your way up to dry fasting from the evening until 12pm the following day)

Today's Notes (Highlights, Thoughts, Feelings, What Could You Improve On?)

"Stay as busy as you can during the daytime. Creating a busy routine makes it easier to manage your diet. Keep setting yourself new tasks/actions in order to keep yourself occupied."

15. Today's Date:

Morning
(work towards continuing your night time dry fast up until at least 12pm)

Afternoon
(get hydrating with fresh fruit or even better slow juiced fruits/berries/melons)

Evening
(aim to wind down to a dry fast by around 6pm to 7pm)

Night
(work your way up to dry fasting from the evening until 12pm the following day)

Today's Notes (Highlights, Thoughts, Feelings, What Could You Improve On?)

"Complete your fruit and fasting routine with a group of friends/family/colleagues so you can all support one another. Make it fun - set challenges - dry fast together and break your fasts together - have weekly catch up sessions."

16. Today's Date:

Morning
(work towards continuing your night time dry fast up until at least 12pm)

Afternoon
(get hydrating with fresh fruit or even better slow juiced fruits/berries/melons)

Evening
(aim to wind down to a dry fast by around 6pm to 7pm)

Night
(work your way up to dry fasting from the evening until 12pm the following day)

Today's Notes (Highlights, Thoughts, Feelings, What Could You Improve On?)

"Monitor your urine regularly in order to ensure your kidneys are filtering. Dry fasting for over 18 hours will increase kidney filtration. You can also drink the juice of slow-juiced citrus fruits (lemons, oranges). Sweating helps too."

17. Today's Date:

Morning
(work towards continuing your night time dry fast up until at least 12pm)

Afternoon
(get hydrating with fresh fruit or even better slow juiced fruits/berries/melons)

Evening
(aim to wind down to a dry fast by around 6pm to 7pm)

Night
(work your way up to dry fasting from the evening until 12pm the following day)

Today's Notes (Highlights, Thoughts, Feelings, What Could You Improve On?)

"Have genuine love and care for yourself. If you are craving junk food, affirm positive inner talk ("I won't feel good after eating junk. I love myself too much to put my body through that. So leave it out!"). You can also take Sea Kelp to reduce any salt cravings."

18. Today's Date:

Morning

(work towards continuing your night time dry fast up until at least 12pm)

Afternoon

(get hydrating with fresh fruit or even better slow juiced fruits/berries/melons)

Evening

(aim to wind down to a dry fast by around 6pm to 7pm)

Night

(work your way up to dry fasting from the evening until 12pm the following day)

Today's Notes (Highlights, Thoughts, Feelings, What Could You Improve On?)

"Feel and note down the difference within yourself as you filter out unwanted acids with this alkaline, water-dense fruits protocol."

19. Today's Date:

Morning

(work towards continuing your night time dry fast up until at least 12pm)

Afternoon

(get hydrating with fresh fruit or even better slow juiced fruits/berries/melons)

Evening

(aim to wind down to a dry fast by around 6pm to 7pm)

Night

(work your way up to dry fasting from the evening until 12pm the following day)

Today's Notes (Highlights, Thoughts, Feelings, What Could You Improve On?)

"Look out for white cloud/sediment (acids) in your urine to confirm that your kidneys are filtering out waste. Urinate in a glass jar - leave for 2 hours to settle before observing."

20. Today's Date:

Morning

(work towards continuing your night time dry fast up until at least 12pm)

Afternoon

(get hydrating with fresh fruit or even better slow juiced fruits/berries/melons)

Evening

(aim to wind down to a dry fast by around 6pm to 7pm)

Night

(work your way up to dry fasting from the evening until 12pm the following day)

Today's Notes (Highlights, Thoughts, Feelings, What Could You Improve On?)

"Infections emerge in an acidic environment. In order to remove infections, you must concentrate on kidney filtration. Use kidney (and adrenal) glandulars and dry fasting to assist."

21. Today's Date:

Morning

(work towards continuing your night time dry fast up until at least 12pm)

Afternoon

(get hydrating with fresh fruit or even better slow juiced fruits/berries/melons)

Evening

(aim to wind down to a dry fast by around 6pm to 7pm)

Night

(work your way up to dry fasting from the evening until 12pm the following day)

Today's Notes (Highlights, Thoughts, Feelings, What Could You Improve On?)

"Any deficiencies that you may have will start to disappear once you have cleansed your congested gut/colon, kidneys and various other eliminative organs."

22. Today's Date:

Morning
(work towards continuing your night time dry fast up until at least 12pm)

Afternoon
(get hydrating with fresh fruit or even better slow juiced fruits/berries/melons)

Evening
(aim to wind down to a dry fast by around 6pm to 7pm)

Night
(work your way up to dry fasting from the evening until 12pm the following day)

Today's Notes (Highlights, Thoughts, Feelings, What Could You Improve On?)

"Dependant on how deeply you detoxify yourself, it is possible to eliminate any genetic weaknesses that you may have inherited. This will require a deep detoxification process which involves juicing your fruits with prolonged periods of dry fasting"

23. Today's Date:

Morning

(work towards continuing your night time dry fast up until at least 12pm)

Afternoon

(get hydrating with fresh fruit or even better slow juiced fruits/berries/melons)

Evening

(aim to wind down to a dry fast by around 6pm to 7pm)

Night

(work your way up to dry fasting from the evening until 12pm the following day)

Today's Notes (Highlights, Thoughts, Feelings, What Could You Improve On?)

"Stay focused on your detoxification for deeper, lasting results. All past injuries / trauma are also repairable for good. Get those old acids out and replace them with a pain-free alkaline environment"

24. Today's Date:

Morning

(work towards continuing your night time dry fast up until at least 12pm)

Afternoon

(get hydrating with fresh fruit or even better slow juiced fruits/berries/melons)

Evening

(aim to wind down to a dry fast by around 6pm to 7pm)

Night

(work your way up to dry fasting from the evening until 12pm the following day)

Today's Notes (Highlights, Thoughts, Feelings, What Could You Improve On?)

*"If you suffer from ongoing sadness /
depression, a deep detox will support your mental health.
You will soon notice a positive change in your mood. Note:
you will need to support your adrenal glands and kidneys
with glandulars and/or herbs"*

25. Today's Date:

Morning
(work towards continuing your night time dry fast up until at least 12pm)

Afternoon
(get hydrating with fresh fruit or even better slow juiced fruits/berries/melons)

Evening
(aim to wind down to a dry fast by around 6pm to 7pm)

Night
(work your way up to dry fasting from the evening until 12pm the following day)

Today's Notes (Highlights, Thoughts, Feelings, What Could You Improve On?)

"Have your fruits/ juices throughout the day - with dry fasting gaps of at least 3 hours in-between each feed. As the evening approaches, start to dry fast fully – from this point on, your body wants to rest and heal."

26. Today's Date:

Morning

(work towards continuing your night time dry fast up until at least 12pm)

Afternoon

(get hydrating with fresh fruit or even better slow juiced fruits/berries/melons)

Evening

(aim to wind down to a dry fast by around 6pm to 7pm)

Night

(work your way up to dry fasting from the evening until 12pm the following day)

Today's Notes (Highlights, Thoughts, Feelings, What Could You Improve On?)

"The kidneys dislike proteins but really appreciate juicy fruits like melons, berries, citrus fruits, pineapples, mangoes, apples, grapes. Witness the difference by replacing cooked foods and protein with fruits. Become the change."

27. Today's Date:

Morning
(work towards continuing your night time dry fast up until at least 12pm)

Afternoon
(get hydrating with fresh fruit or even better slow juiced fruits/berries/melons)

Evening
(aim to wind down to a dry fast by around 6pm to 7pm)

Night
(work your way up to dry fasting from the evening until 12pm the following day)

Today's Notes (Highlights, Thoughts, Feelings, What Could You Improve On?)

"Healing is very easy. There's no need to complicate it. Keep everything simple and you will see results. Concentrate on improving your level of health to a point where dis-ease is dissolved"

28. Today's Date:

Morning
(work towards continuing your night time dry fast up until at least 12pm)

Afternoon
(get hydrating with fresh fruit or even better slow juiced fruits/berries/melons)

Evening
(aim to wind down to a dry fast by around 6pm to 7pm)

Night
(work your way up to dry fasting from the evening until 12pm the following day)

Today's Notes (Highlights, Thoughts, Feelings, What Could You Improve On?)

"Keep your body in an alkaline and hydrated state as this is where regeneration takes place - and disease cannot continue to exist. You can achieve this through a raw fruits and vegetables diet (find your balance between the two)"

29. Today's Date:

Morning
(work towards continuing your night time dry fast up until at least 12pm)

Afternoon
(get hydrating with fresh fruit or even better slow juiced fruits/berries/melons)

Evening
(aim to wind down to a dry fast by around 6pm to 7pm)

Night
(work your way up to dry fasting from the evening until 12pm the following day)

Today's Notes (Highlights, Thoughts, Feelings, What Could You Improve On?)

"A daily enema with boiled water (cooled down) will support your detox greatly. Do not however become dependant on enemas, so after the initial week, start to wean yourself off."

30. Today's Date:

Morning
(work towards continuing your night time dry fast up until at least 12pm)

Afternoon
(get hydrating with fresh fruit or even better slow juiced fruits/berries/melons)

Evening
(aim to wind down to a dry fast by around 6pm to 7pm)

Night
(work your way up to dry fasting from the evening until 12pm the following day)

Today's Notes (Highlights, Thoughts, Feelings, What Could You Improve On?)

"Have your iris' read by an iridologist that works with Dr Bernard Jensen's system. An Iris Diagnosis will offer you information on specific areas of weakness that you can focus on"

www.ingramcontent.com/pod-product-compliance
Lightning Source LLC
Chambersburg PA
CBHW031204020426
42333CB00013B/793